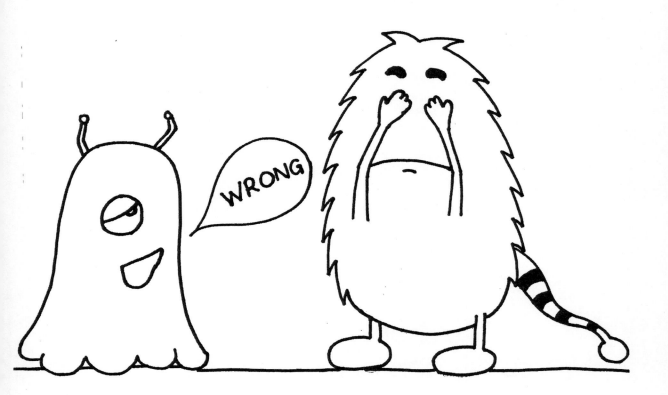

Sometimes I say and do things I don't even know are wrong until someone tells me.

I don't like that.
I don't like people to see how bad I am and how wrong I get everything.

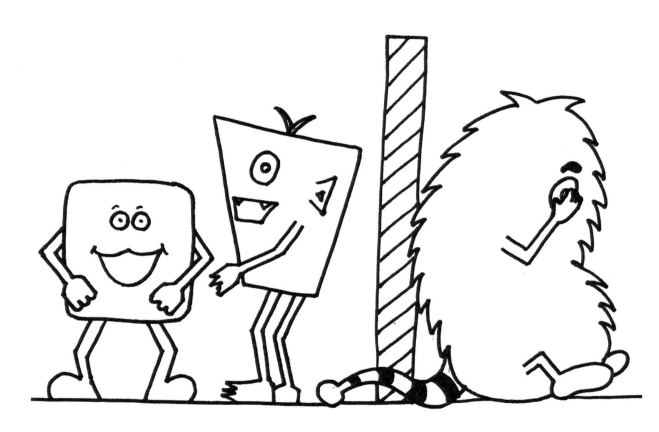

Sometimes I Get Things Wrong.

Worrying William's Story.

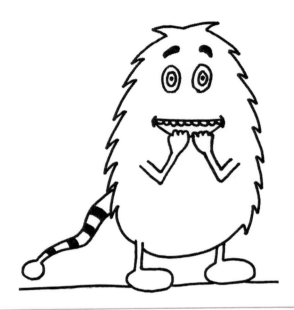

This book belongs to:

This is your book.

Draw in it. Doodle over it. Write within it. Colour in the lines or go over them.

It's totally up to you.

Published by
Belong Therapeutic Support
in Solihull, UK
www.belongts.com
www.belong-blog.com

Text copyright F Newood 2017
Illustrations copyright G Newood 2017
First Published 2017

This book is a work of fiction. Names, characters, businesses, organisations, places and events are a product of the author's imagination or are used factiously. Any resemblance to actual persons, living or dead, events or locales is entirely coincidental.

ISBN: 978-0-9926629-3-6

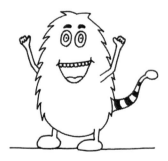

This book is dedicated to
Jane Foulkes.
Thank you for helping us every time
we've got things wrong.
Love Fi and Gail.

Sometimes I Get Things Wrong.

Worrying William's Story.

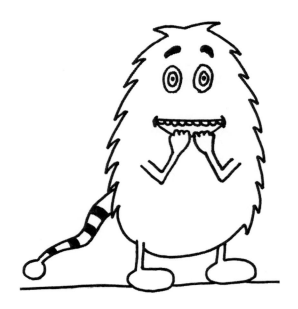

How Worrying William
Deals With Shame.

Written by Fi Newood
Illustrated by Gail Newood

Sometimes I get things wrong.

Actually, I feel like I get a lot of things wrong a lot of the time.

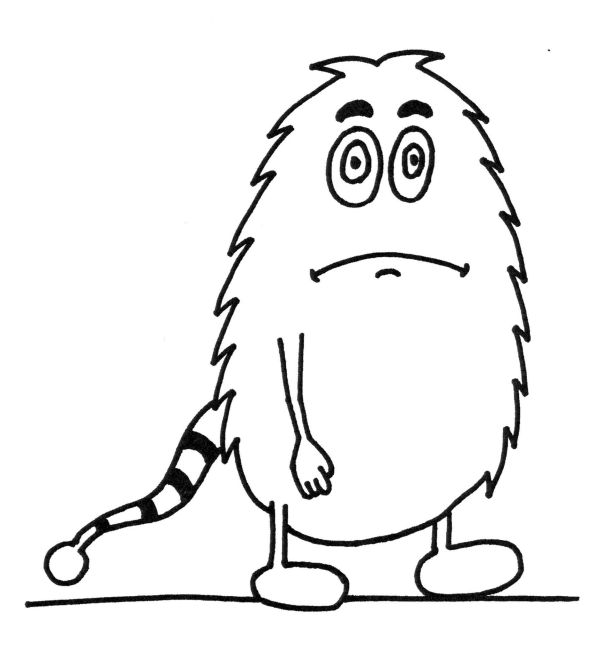

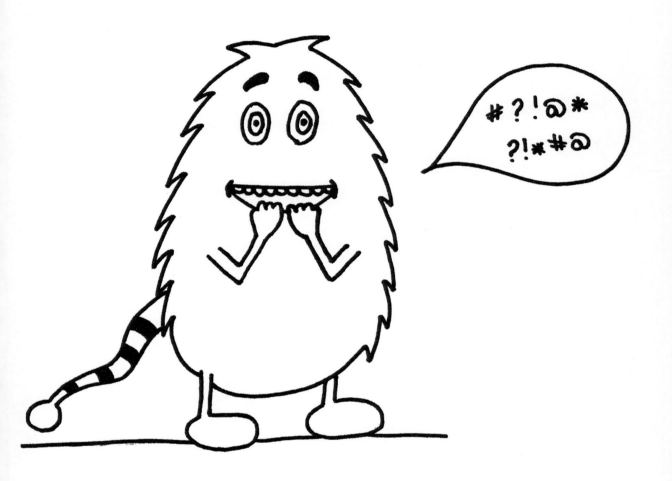

Sometimes I say things and then wish
I hadn't said them.

Sometimes I do things and then wish I hadn't done them.

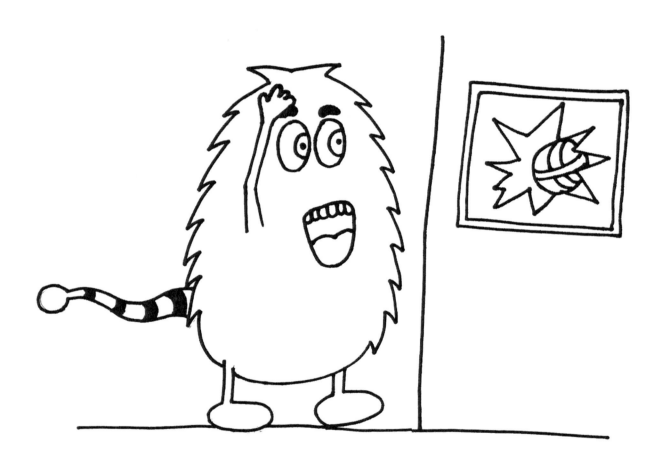

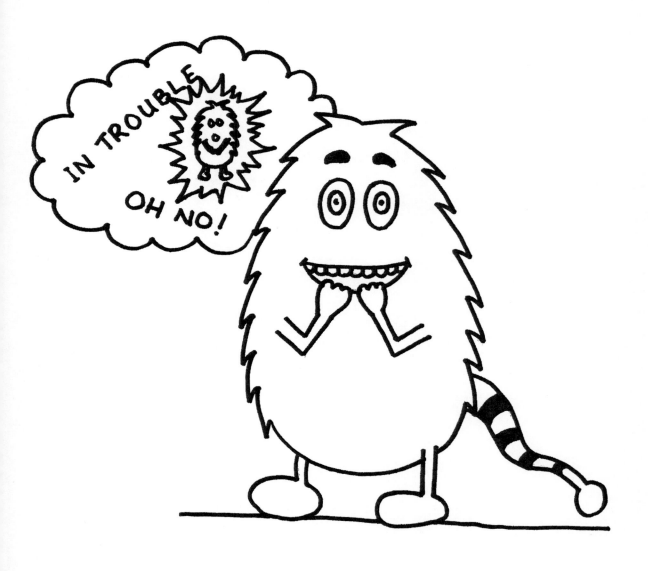

I also don't like it when people tell me off because I worry what might happen next.

So I have lots of ways of trying to make sure that no-one finds out if I've done something wrong.

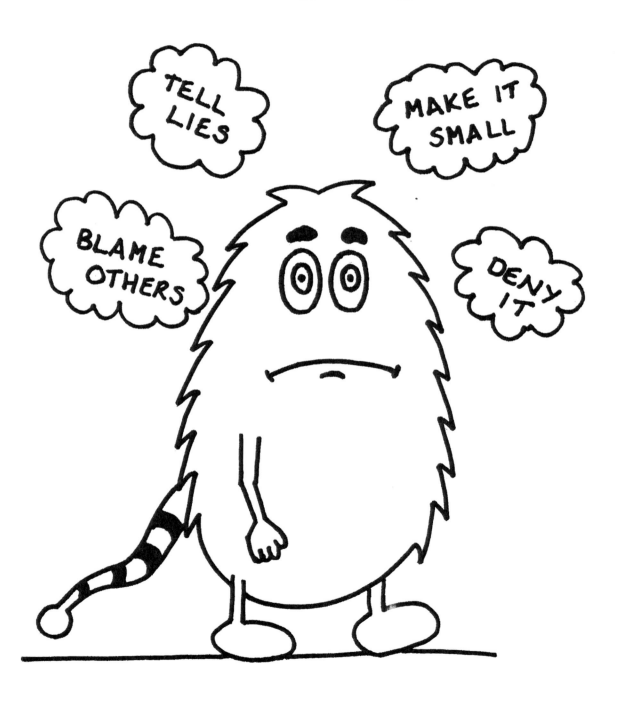

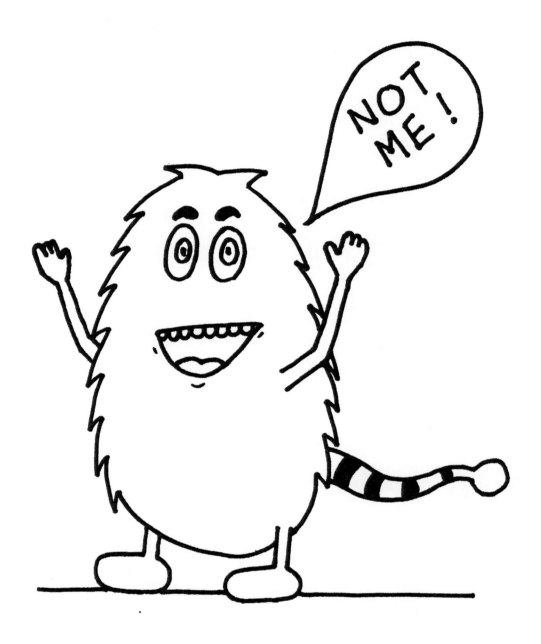

Sometimes I deny it.
I say "I didn't do it" even though I
did.

Sometimes I lie.
I say "I wasn't even there!" when really I was.

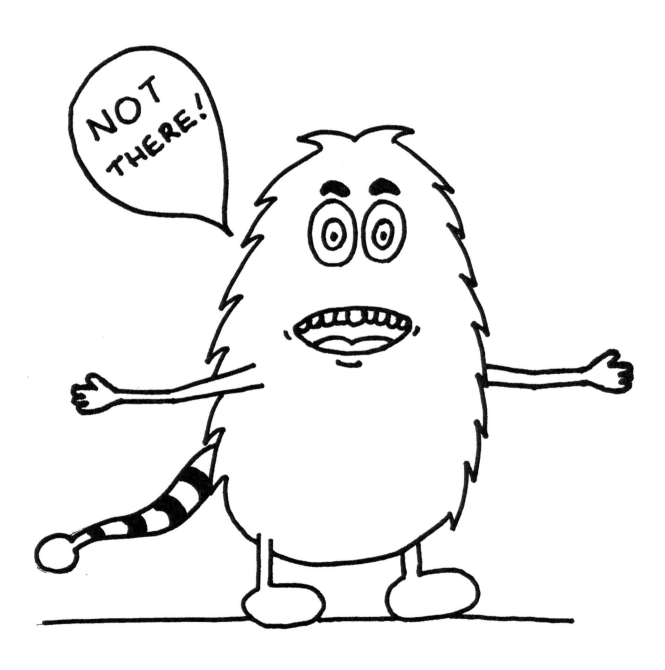

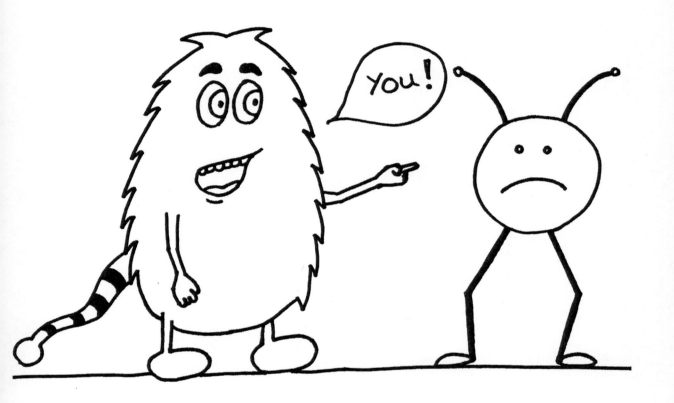

Sometimes I blame others.
I say "It was her!" when really it was me.

When they already know it was me I worry about getting in big, big trouble. So I tell them it was only a little thing really, even though it wasn't.

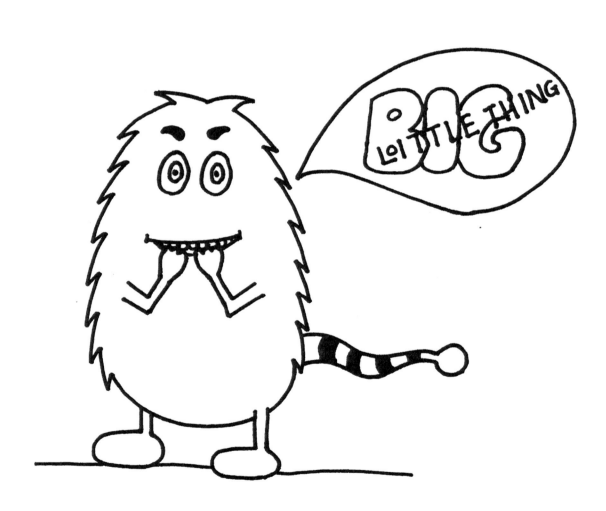

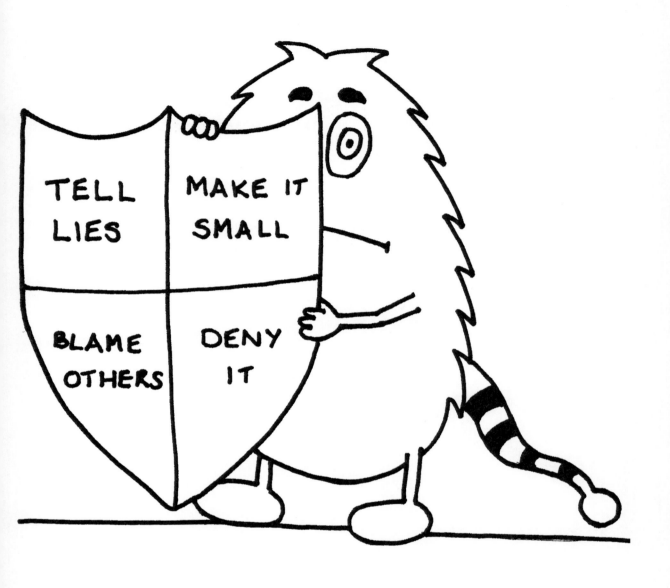

All these things I say are like a shield
I use to stop people from seeing how
bad I am or being cross with me.

The shield doesn't always work. In fact, it doesn't work a lot of the time and that makes me feel really, really bad about myself and really, really angry.

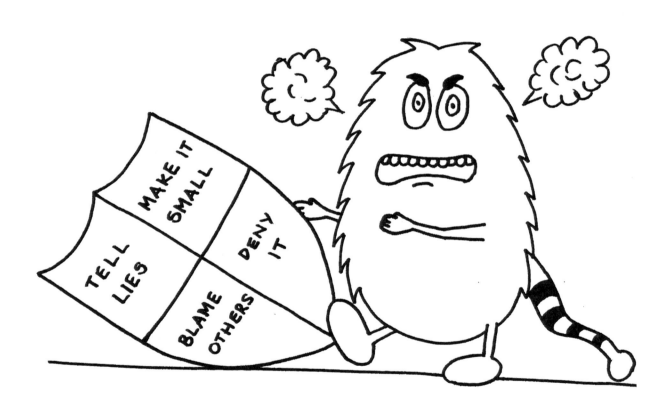

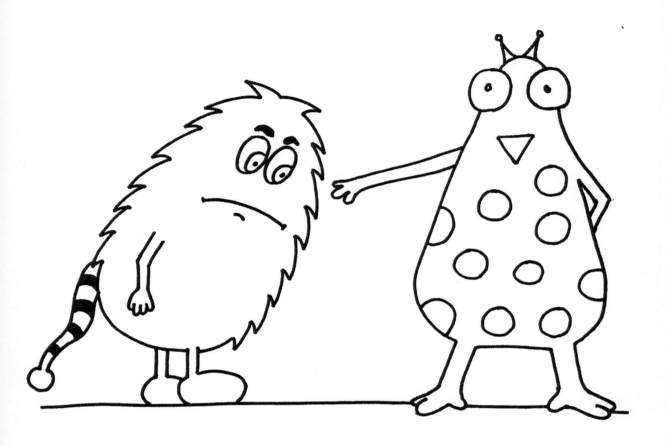

I don't like those feelings so the last time I did something wrong, I did something brave. I told a helpful adult what I had done and how I was feeling.

I thought she was going to be very, very cross with me but she wasn't. She told me that it was ok to get things wrong. She said that everybody does this sometimes. She said that even good people make bad choices. She said that I was a good person, but I don't know if I can believe that.

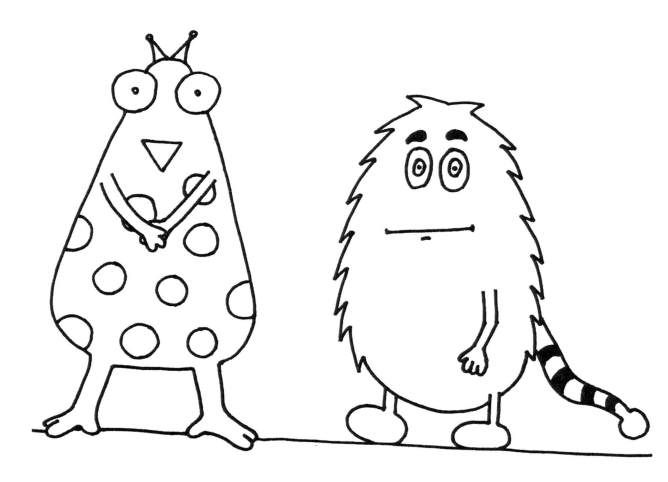

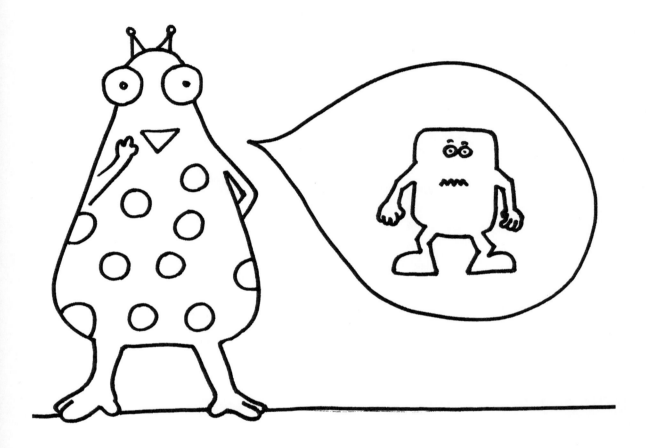

She told me that there are lots of reasons why people make bad choices. Sometimes people do the wrong thing because they are feeling scared or anxious.

Sometimes people do the wrong thing because they worry what will happen if they don't.

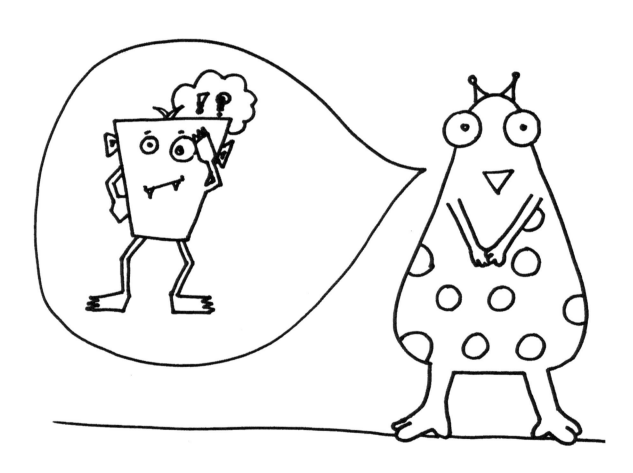

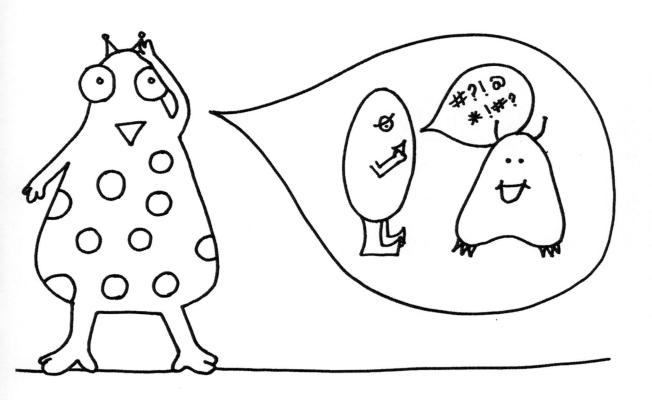

Sometimes people make poor choices
because someone else has taught
them to do that.

And sometimes people don't even know that their choices are wrong.

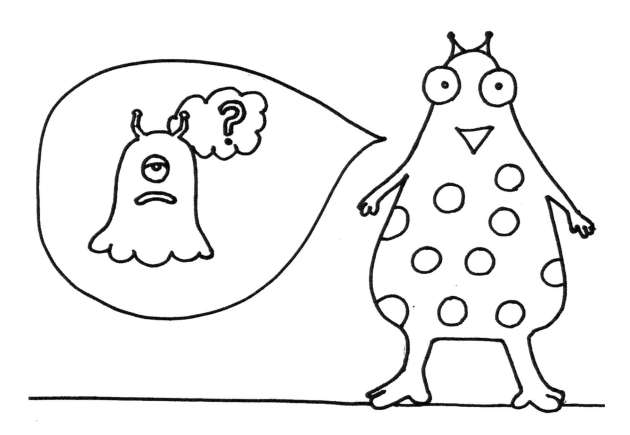

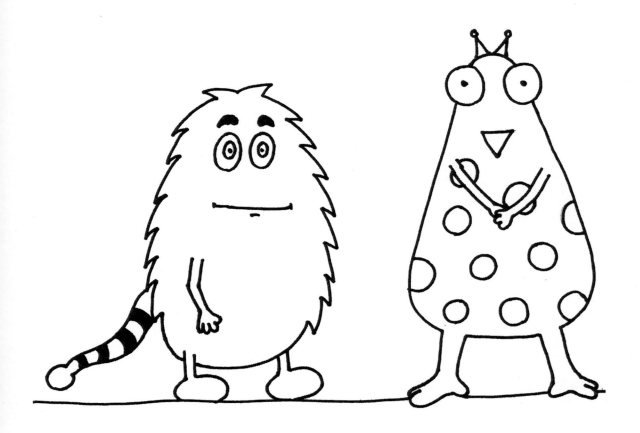

"No-one is perfect" she said. We all
have parts of ourselves that make
mistakes or poor choices. That
doesn't make us 'bad', it makes us just
like everyone else. She said that even
she got things wrong sometimes.

It wasn't easy being brave but I did feel a bit better after I talked to her.

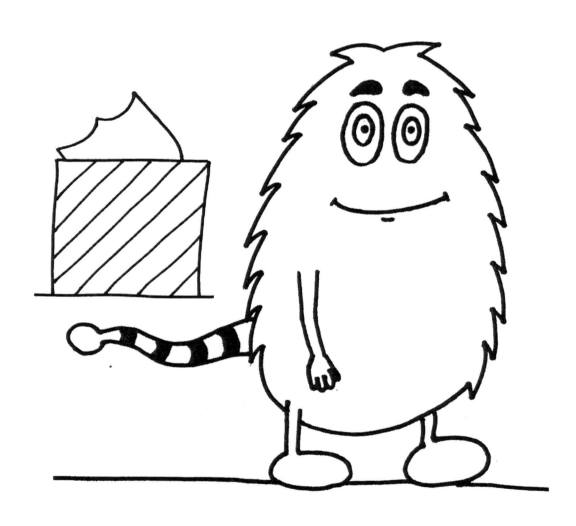

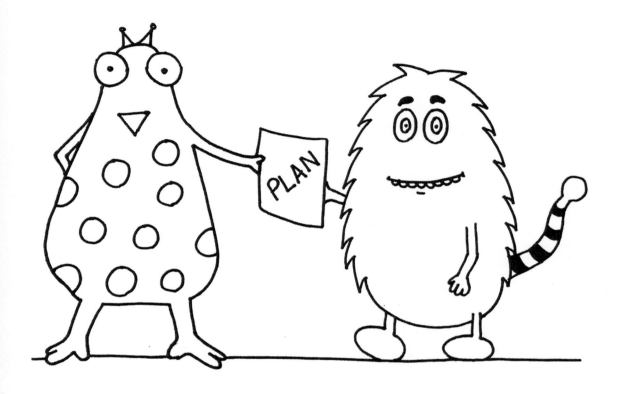

We were even able to come up with a plan for what I could do the next time I got something wrong. She said she would help me and I know she really wants to.

So when I make poor choices in the future I know I need to ask an adult to help me because otherwise I really will be getting something wrong.

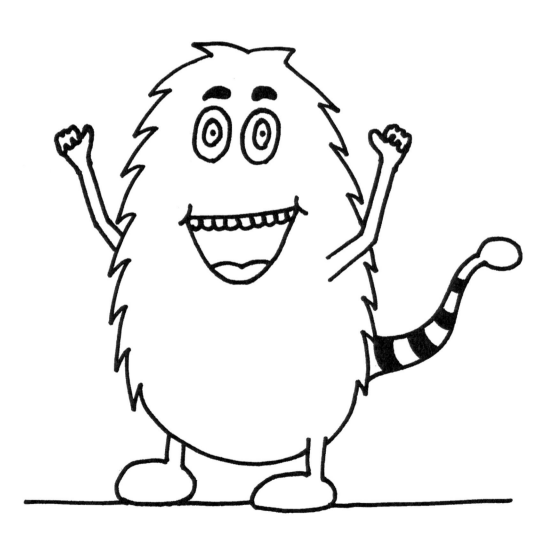

The End.

Our Other Books

Sometimes I Run

A book for young people who want to run away when things get difficult.

Why Can't I Do That?

A book for young people who feel different to others.

Sometimes I Fight

A book for young people who fight and argue when things get difficult

I Can't Do This!

A book foster and adoptive parents who are finding things hard.